Berberine

Users Guide on Cancer Control, Health Benefits of Berberine on Human, Side Effects, Uses and Recommendation on Berberine. (Sex Drive and Women Dillodo)

Dionisia Onio

Table of Contents

INTRODUCTION

Heart disease, cancer, Alzheimer's disease and diabetes are all leading causes of death in the world. Combined, these conditions kill over 1.25 million Americans annually not to talk of the numbers people across the globe. Fortunately, there's a solution that addresses all of these ailments naturally - berberine. This multifaceted plant extract that you've probably never heard of could easily increase longevity, improve your quality of life and help you reduce or eliminate the need for pharmaceutical medications.

Learn how Berberine can boost your overall health. Learning about ways that you can supplement a healthy diet is a great step in the right direction towards a healthier you!

CHAPTER 1

BERBERINE

Berberine is a bioactive compound that can be extracted from numerous plants, consisting of a collection of shrubs called ***Berberis***.

Technically, it belongs to a class of compounds called alkaloids. It has a yellow color, and has regularly been used as a dye.

Berberine has a long history of use in traditional Chinese medicine, which turns out to be used to deal with diverse ailments.

Now, modern-day science has showed that it has awesome benefits for numerous special health issues.

A compound called *Berberine* is one of the best herbal dietary (natural) supplements to be had.

It has very incredible health benefits, and impacts your body at the molecular level.

Berberine has been shown to decrease blood sugar, cause weight loss and enhance coronary heart health, to call a few.

It is one of the few supplements shown to be as powerful as a pharmaceutical drug.

Berberine comes to us from china and India, where it became first utilized in traditional Chinese and Ayurvedic drugs. Berberine is a natural alkaloid located in a wide variety of traditional herbs, consisting of goldenseal, barberry, goldthread, oregon grape, tree turmeric and phellodendron.

Within this plant, the berberine alkaloid can also be discovered in the stem bark, roots and rhizomes (rootlike subterranean stems) of the plant.

Berberine extracts are usually cheaper, secure and well-known for their vast antibacterial activities — and can certainly help in dealing (treating) with situations naturally without always resorting to antibiotics, as currently we've got a completely critical and growing problem of antibiotic resistance in majority of the world.

Berberine has been proven to have many different pharmacological effects along with being antimicrobial, anti-tumor, anti-inflammatory and blood glucose–lowering.

Nutritional Background of Berberine

Berberine is an alkaloid, which is defined as a category of organic compounds of plant origin containing ordinarily simple nitrogen atoms which have suggested physiological actions on human beings. There is a sturdy amount of research on berberine that has been performed thus far with repeated double-blind clinical trials.

Findings of those research have proven definitive or probably advantages for a totally extensive range of serious health ailments, inclusive of:

- Anti-growing older

- Diabetes

- Gastrointestinal infections

- Coronary heart disease

- High cholesterol

- Hypertension (high blood pressure)

- Immune challenges

- Joint problems

- Low bone density

- Weight control

What Herbs Are High in Berberine?

Herbal supplement sales have steadily increased over the past few years; however, one botanical you won't find among the bestsellers is *Berberine*. In reality, if you can find it at all, it's possibly in products containing berberine-rich herbs which includes goldenseal, Oregon grape, barberry, and goldthread (Coptis chinensis), aimed at curtailing bacterial, viral, fungal, yeast, and parasitic infections.

That's about to change. This plant alkaloid, revered in traditional Chinese language and Ayurvedic medicine but in large part neglected somewhere else, is poised to turn out to be one in every of our most effective natural healing procedures for preventing and treating diabetes and cardiovascular disease, facilitating weight loss, preventing most cancers, and perhaps even staving off dementia and the ravages of getting old.

CHAPTER 2

7 Health Benefits of Berberine

Diabetes

As the rate of diabetes is rising steadily round the world, studies showed that berberine deserves a place amongst different natural treatments for diabetes. At some point of one study, berberine was found to lower blood glucose, supporting to prevent and deal with Type 2 diabetes and its complications, including diabetic cardiovascular ailment and diabetic neuropathies.

One of the maximum marvelous studies on berberine compared taking 500 milligrams of the compound two to 3 times daily for 3 months with taking the common diabetes drug *metformin*. Berberine was capable of controlling blood sugar and lipid metabolism as efficiently as metformin, with researchers describing berberine as a "effective oral hypoglycemic agent."

Additional studies have also indicated that berberine improves glucose and lipid metabolism disorders. More mainly, an examine published in proof-based complementary and alternative medicine that berberine can improve insulin sensitivity by way of adjusting adipokine secretion.

High Cholesterol

There is early evidence which shows that berberine can help lower high levels of cholesterol. A Metabolism study showed that berberine decreased serum cholesterol along with triglyceride levels. While *dangerous statin therapy* (the conventional pharmaceutical treatment of high cholesterol) increases the risk for Type 2 diabetes, among other risks, berberine likely has the opposite effect.

A separate study discovered that the mixed administration of red yeast rice (famous for its ability to naturally decrease cholesterol) and berberine may offer a broader range of cholesterol protection with a lower risk of great unfavorable outcomes compared with prescription statin therapy. Berberine has been shown to lower abnormally excessive concentrations of fats and lipids in the blood with the aid of promoting the excretion of cholesterol from the liver and inhibiting the intestinal absorption of cholesterol.

Obesity

Because of extreme adverse effect and the confined effectiveness of currently available pharmaceutical treatment options for weight problems (obesity), many research efforts have been focusing at the creation of natural remedies for weight problems — inclusive of anti-obesity drugs from natural products.

Along those lines, berberine is one of the few compounds regarded to activate adenosine monophosphate-activated protein kinase or AMPK. AMPK is an enzyme inside the human body's cells, which is frequently known as a "metabolic master switch" since it plays a critical role in regulating metabolism. AMPK activation boosts fat burning inside the mitochondria. Studies have validated that berberine prevented fat accumulation in the human body.

In a single pilot study published in phytomedicine, obese human subjects (Caucasian) had been given 500 milligrams of berberine orally 3 times in step with day for a total of 12 weeks. The efficacy and safety of berberine treatment was determined via measurements of body weight, complete metabolic panel, blood lipid and hormone levels, expression levels of inflammatory elements, complete blood count, and electrocardiograph. Overall, this study was demonstrated that berberine is a potent lipid-lowering compound with a mild weight loss effect.

Alzheimer's Disease

Studies have evaluated the therapeutic potential of berberine in opposition to neurodegenerative diseases like alzheimer's disease, parkinson's disease and trauma-induced neurodegeneration. One study discovered that there are a couple of advantageous consequences of berberine, a number of which enhances neuroprotective factors/pathways and others that counteract neurodegeneration.

The promising results seen up till now offer a convincing and good sized basis to support further clinical exploration and development of the therapeutic potential of berberine in opposition to neurodegenerative diseases.

Small Intestinal Bacterial Overgrowth or SIBO

Patients who are afflicted by small intestine bacterial overgrowth (SIBO) symptoms have excessive bacteria in their small intestines. Present conventional remedy of SIBO is limited to oral antibiotics with inconsistent achievement. More and more, people who are affected by SIBO are inquisitive about the usage of complementary and alternative therapies for their gastrointestinal health.

The goal of one study published by Global Advances in Health and Medicine was to determine the remission rate of SIBO the usage of an antibiotic as opposed to an herbal remedy. It determined that the herbal treatment, which included berberine, worked just as well as antibiotic treatment and was equally secure.

Heart Health

Part of berberine's tremendous positive impact on heart healthy likely stems from the compound's ability to help hold blood sugar levels and obesity in check, both of which could enhance the risk of coronary heart disease. Berberine also stimulates the release of nitric oxide (NO), a signaling molecule that relaxes the arteries, increases blood flow, lowers blood pressure and protects against arteriosclerosis.

In research published by the University of Maryland Medical Centre, people who took berberine for eight weeks had better coronary heart function and have higher capability of performing exercise than individuals who took a placebo. The recommended dosage from this study was 300 to 500 milligrams, four times per day. The cardiovascular effects of berberine also advise on its possible clinical usefulness in the treatment of arrhythmias and heart failure.

Lung Health

Berberine's potent anti-inflammatory properties are also awesome for lung health. Berberine has been proven to reduce the impact of cigarette smoke-induced acute lung inflammation.

In a study published in the journal inflammation, mice were exposed to cigarette smoke to cause acute lung injury and had been then given (50 mg/kg, intragastrically). Upon examination of lung tissues, it turns out that cigarette smoke brought about inflammation of the lung's alveoli together with cellular edema or abnormal fluid retention. However, pretreatment with berberine substantially lessened lung inflammation and ameliorated cigarette smoke-brought about acute lung injury through its anti-inflammatory activity.

CHAPTER 3

Berberine As a Control to Cancer

Latest research indicates that berberine also has a role in most cancers' prevention and treatment, as it inhibits the growth of most cancers' cells, induces apoptosis (tumor cell death), curbs the improvement of blood vessels that feed tumors, and help prevent metastasis.

Although most of the research is in animal models of human cancers, it is quite compelling. In a study of breast cancer, as an instance, it stopped cell cycle growth more effectively than doxorubicin, a commonly used drug, and has proven to be more effective against a variety of tumor types.

Berberine is nowhere close to being an accepted cancer treatment, however because this natural compound enhances sensitivity to chemotherapy and radiation, hence improving their efficacy, it ought to be taken into consideration as an adjunct therapy.

Possible Side Effects of Berberine

If you have a clinical circumstance or are on any medications consisting of antibiotics, then it is miles encouraged that you speak for your health practitioner earlier than taking berberine. This is most essential in case you are presently taking blood sugar–lowering medication.

As far as berberine can lower blood sugar, diabetics who're controlling their blood sugar with insulin or other medications have to use caution while using berberine to avoid dangerously low blood sugar levels. People with low blood pressure should be cautious while using berberine on the grounds that it may naturally lower blood pressure. Pregnant and nursing girls should not take berberine.

Overall, berberine has an outstanding safety profile. The principal side effects are associated with digestion and are minor, as there are some reports of cramping, diarrhea, flatulence, constipation and stomach pain. Once more, by sticking with recommended smaller dosages — spread out through your day and after meals — these possible minor negative side effects can be prevented all together.

Is Berberine Better Than Metformin?

Berberine has been on my radar for years for fighting infections and boosting intestinal health, but i was pleasantly surprised when I came across a study demonstrating its capability to lower blood sugar—and astonished to realize that it worked as well as metformin

(Glucophage), the most famous drug for Type 2 diabetes!

In a medical trial published in metabolism, people with newly diagnosed Type 2 diabetes have been randomly divided into two and assigned to take metformin or berberine. Improvements were cited the very first week, and at the study's conclusion, the average blood sugar and hemoglobin A1c levels drastically reduced in each group. Remarkably, berberine was every bit as powerful as metformin. The 2 had "identical effect[s] in the regulation of glucose metabolism."

Lipids, Blood Pressure, and Weight

Reducing blood sugar is just one major thing in every berberine's strengths. Another study, a randomized, placebo-controlled trial, involved patients who have been recently diagnosed with diabetes and dyslipidemia (cholesterol/triglyceride abnormalities) but hadn't but began on drugs. They had been informed to take either 500 mg of berberine or a placebo tablet two times a day.

Like in the preceding study, 3 months of berberine supplementation led to blood sugar improvements that were "completely similar with that of existing pharmacologic products used in treatment of Type 2 diabetes."

However, berberine did something diabetes drugs cannot do. It decreased triglycerides by 35.9%, LDL cholesterol by 21 percent, and general cholesterol by 18 percent, in comparison to minimum declines in cholesterol and an increase in triglycerides in the control group. Moreover, the group taking berberine had lower blood pressure (average drop of 7/5 mm Hg systolic/diastolic) and modest weight and abdominal fat loss.

Is Berberine Too Good to Be True?

How can one plant extract have a lot of these numerous benefits? It sounds too good to be real—until you realize that berberine targets a completely fundamental and historical regulator of metabolism found in all animals and plants referred to as AMP-activated protein kinase (AMPK).

Activated by reduced ATP (energy) production, AMPK turns on a couple of protective metabolic pathways to ensure survival in time of stress. I've written before about the profound benefits of calorie restriction. Now we realize that a number one motive lowering food consumption prevents disease and extends life span is because it revs up AMPK activity.

AMPK stimulates the uptake of glucose into the cells, improves insulin sensitivity, and reduces glucose production inside the liver, which is in overdrive in

24

patients with diabetes. It slows the release of unfastened fatty acids, which lowers lipid levels and prevents harmful fats deposition, and boosts fat burning in the mitochondria. It additionally stimulates the discharge of nitric oxide (NO), a signaling molecule that relaxes the arteries, increases blood float and lowers blood pressure, and protects against atherosclerosis. Similarly, it inhibits mTORC1, a pathway that promotes cellular proliferation and inhibits apoptosis, which seems to be important to its anti-cancer's effects.

Drugs or Berberine?

Folks, what we've got here is safe, less expensive, natural complement that mirrors the effects of the top-selling diabetes drug and lowers lipids, blood pressure, and weight and fights most cancers. Yet hardly anyone knows about it!

Mark my words, you may be hearing a lot, plenty and more about AMPK activation in the nearest future—most in all likelihood in the promotion of medicine such as metformin, which also targets AMPK and is being studied as a treatment for a huge variety of condition.

I'll put my money on berberine any day. Metformin can be the most secure diabetes drug; however, it still has an extended list of side effects.

Most importantly, berberine does things that drug producers handiest desire any single drug could do. In addition to the above benefits, studies show that berberine improves bone density and preserves cartilage, protects against acute brain damage and neurodegenerative problems, and might play a role in warding off dementia and Alzheimer's disease. And because it mimics the effects of calorie limit, i am expecting and predict that berberine may be the next big thing in anti-growing older.

Recommendation

- Berberine is an excellent primary or adjunct therapy for diabetes, cardiovascular concern, most cancers and immune challenges, intestinal infections, and as a common health supplement.

- The standard dose is 500mg 2–3 times a day. Although it is commonly nicely tolerated, berberine can cause constipation, which commonly clears up over time or with a reduction in dosage.

CHAPTER 4

Where to Find Berberine & How to Use it

Berberine can be found in supplement form online or in maximum health food stores. Be cautious in order not to confuse berberine with piperine (black pepper extract), berberrubine (a metabolite) or berberol (a logo call mixture of tree turmeric and milk thistle).

Considering that berberine have a short half-life, you generally need to take this supplement three times a day so as to keep stable levels in your blood. Many research use dosages of 900 to at least 1,500 milligrams per day. It's most commonly recommended to take 500 milligrams, three times per day for a complete 1,500 milligrams in a day.

Berberine should be taken with a meal, or immediately after the meal, to take advantage of the blood glucose and lipid spike that incorporates consuming a meal. High doses of berberine taken acutely may cause belly upset, cramping and/or diarrhea, which is another precise motive to take berberine in multiple doses at some point of the day.

You can work with a natural health care practitioner to decide the dose of berberine that works best for you.

Interesting Facts about Berberine

Berberine has been a revered plant alkaloid in traditional Chinese and Ayurvedic medicinal drug for centuries. Berberine is the main active thing of an historic Chinese herb Coptis Chinensis French, which has been used to naturally treat diabetes for hundreds of years. Berberine has additionally been used to deal with bacterial gastroenteritis, diarrhea and other digestive diseases for more than 1,000 years.

There is increasing studies on the regulation of cancer cell metabolism by berberine hydrochloride. Berberine's anticancer activity, particularly inhibiting growth and proliferation of cancer cells, make it likely to end up a natural component of the nanoparticulate delivery systems used for most cancers therapy. Berberine has also been proven to have a probable potential role in osteoporosis treatment and prevention.

Some people apply berberine directly to the pores and skin to treat burns and also to the attention to treat bacterial infections, like trachoma, that frequently causes blindness. Berberine has been shown to be effective towards a huge range of bacteria, protozoa and fungi. Animal studies have also proven that berberine might also help combat depression.

Recommendations

1) Diabetes: The Complete Guide on Type 1 & Type 2 Diabetes, Signs, Causes and Treatments. A Long-Lasting Solution to Diabetes Mellitus with the Help of Medication, Self-Monitoring and Healthy Diets.

   http://getBook.at/diabetes

2) Diabetes Management: Complete Guide and A Long-Lasting Solution to Diabetes Mellitus with the Help of Medication, Self-Monitoring and Healthy Diets.

   http://getBook.at/Diabetesmanagement

3) Reverse Diabetes: Step By Step Guide On How To Prevent Diabetes Mellitus & Insipidus With The Help Of Insulin, Healthy Diet. A Better

Approach to cure Hypoglycemia and Hyperglycemia.

http://getBook.at/Reversediabetes

4) Diabetes Control: The Complete Guide on Type 1 & Type 2 Diabetes, Pre-Diabetes, Gestational Diabetes, Signs and Symptoms, Causes and Treatments.

http://getBook.at/Diabetescontrol

5) How and Where to Buy Viagra Online Safely, Legally and Cheap: The Secret Behind How to Buy Viagra Online Safely Without A Prescription (With List Of Best Place To Buy Viagra Online)

http://getbook.at/viagraonline

6) Viagra & Sildenafil: Uses, Dosage, Side Effects and Risks Information: The Secret Guide Behind

How to Buy Viagra Online Safely, Cheap and Legally (With Best Online Pharmacy for Generic Viagra)

http://getBook.at/viagra

7) Erectile Dysfunction (ED): Symptoms & Causes, Diagnosis, Treatment Online, And More Using Viagra Without a Prescription (Including Where to Buy Viagra, Cialis, Levitra etc. Drugs Cheap & Safely Online

http://getBook.at/erectile

8) Innovative Visualisation: The Power of Mind Perception -- GET MORE DONE THROUGH MIND MANIPULATION, INCENTIVES, PSYCH TRICKS AND MORE

http://getBook.at/innovative

9) <u>Natural Healing and Remedies Cyclopedia</u>:
Complete solution with herbal medicine, Essential
oils natural remedies and natural cure to various
illness. (The answer to prayer for healing)
<u>http://getBook.at/naturalhealing</u>

10) <u>100 BEST CAT WELLNESS FOOD, DIET &</u>
<u>RECIPES</u>: The hidden healing power diet for cat
kidney problems, cat weight-loss, & pregnant cat
diet; including recipes for all cat diseases and
illness <u>http://myBook.to/catfood</u>

11) <u>The Brain, Mind and Memory Therapy:</u> The
Science of embracing Change, Boosting Brain
Power, Increasing Your Energy and Mental
Strength.
<u>http://getBook.at/brainbook</u>

12) **What Wikipedia Can't Tell You About Achieving Your Goals**: Why your objective setting never works out the way you plan

http://getBook.at/wikipedia

13) **The First Year From Childbirth and beyond:** Inside-out Information on what to expect the first year and beyond early childhood for mothers and fathers made simple

http://getBook.at/childbirth

We love Testimonies, and we want to know how thus our publications have been of immense help to you. And please consider writing to us at www.engolee.com

Follow us on Social media at:

Website: www.engolee.com

Facebook Page: www.facebook.com/engolee

Twitter Page: www.twitter.com/engolee

About the Author

Dionisia Onio is an Health Researcher from Italy who has developed a series of fabulous and highly effective healthful strategies. She applies her knowledge and astonishing perception to analyze the background and underlying causes of various diseases and health related problems affecting people in the world and then designs individualized and totally effective strategies to attain the desired results in solving human related problem with diseases.

Acknowledgments

The Glory of this book success goes to God Almighty and my beautiful Family, Fans, Readers & well-wishers, Customers and Friends for their endless support and encouragements.